ESSENTIAL OIL
MAKE&TAKES
OVER 70 DIY PROJECTS AND RECIPES
SECOND EDITION

JEN O'SULLIVAN

ESSENTIAL OIL MAKE & TAKES *by Jen O'Sullivan*
Second Edition Copyright ©2020 by Jen O'Sullivan
First Edition Copyright ©2017 by Jen O'Sullivan
www.31oils.com

Cover and Interior Design by Jen O'Sullivan
Cover Photo by J. Chizhe

All rights reserved. No part of this book may be reproduced, distributed, or transmitted in any form or by any means, electronic or mechanical, including online posting, photocopying, recording, or by any information storage and retrieval system, without the prior written consent from the author. Single recipe quotes are allowed with book name and author credit.

ISBN: 978-1-7344993-5-3

Printed in the United States of America

Second Edition November 2020

ESSENTIAL OIL MAKE & TAKES *by Jen O'Sullivan*

CONTENTS

4 INTRODUCTION
6 THE RECIPES
6 Baby Bottom Paste
6 Baby Gum Soothing Serum
7 Baby Scalp Scrub & Serum
8 Bath Salts
9 Bath Soak (Oatmeal)
9 Bikini Line Serum
10 Body Sugar Scrub
11 Body Wash
11 Bubble Bath
12 Car Vent Diffuser
13 Cool-Down Spray
13 Critter Spray
14 Face Cleanser
15 Face Exfoliator
16 Eye Serum
16 Face Serum (All Skin Types)
17 Face Serum (Blemish Support)
17 Face Toner Spray
18 Fingernail Support
18 Fizzies (Bath Bombs)
19 Fragrance
20 Hand Lotion
21 Hand Soap (Foaming)
21 Hand Scrubbing Balls
22 Hair Conditioning Rinse
22 Hair Deep Cleanser
23 Hair Deep Conditioner
24 Hair Detangling Spray
24 Hair Detangling Spray (Easy)
25 Hair Dry Shampoo
26 Hair Follicle Spray
27 Hair Serum
27 Hair Shampoo
28 Hair Split End Spray
28 Hair Shine Spray
29 Heel and Foot Cream

Home: Candles 30
Home: Degreaser 31
Home: Drawer Sachets 31
Home: Room Freshener 32
Home: Window Cleaner 32
Hydrosol 33
Lip Balm 34
Lip Scrub 34
Lucy Libido's Skinamint 35
Makeup Removing Pads 35
Manly Aftershave 36
Manly Beard Balm 36
Manly Beard Oil 37
Manly Muscle Support 37
Mouthwash 38
Nipple Butter 39
Potty-pourri Spray 39
Rollerballs 40
Scalp Serum Mask 41
Scalp Spray 41
Sunscreen 42
Toenail Support 43
Tooth Polish 43
Underarm Support 44
Underarm Support (Easy) 44
Whipped Body Butter 45

LABELS 46
HOLIDAY PARTY 48
100 GIFTS 49
FINAL THOUGHTS 54
INGREDIENT LIST 56
RESOURCES 57
EQUIPMENT LIST 57
SUPPLY LIST 57
HOW TO HOST A PARTY 58
MAKE & TAKE PARTY SCRIPT 60
ADDITIONAL EDUCATION 62
AUTHOR BIOGRAPHY 63

INTRODUCTION

When you find natural solutions and life hacks to everyday needs, it is fun to start making your own home-made personal care products that support health rather than deteriorate it. Most of us spend over half of our lives in our home. We sleep for 25-33% of our lives, the other percent is taken up by when we eat breakfast and dinner, relax and play with family, all inside or around our home. Did you know that over half of the women who work from home get some sort of disease related to the chemicals in their home? A 15 year study done by the Environmental Protection Agency showed that "Stay at home moms and women who work from home are 54% more likely to die from cancer than women who don't work from home." Let that sink in for a moment. How do you think your pets are fairing if they are in your home for the majority of their lives?

It's quite shocking when you start to realize it's your home that may be killing you. The very sanctuary of rest and restoration is the place that is causing your disease and illness. When it comes to all of these synthetic toxins, often times the damage is done to you. Consider your own health. You may be unable to focus or be your best self because you are depressed, tired all of the time, not sleeping well, gaining weight, feeling overwhelmed, out of control, feeling anxious, having a hard time focusing, experiencing erratic emotions, or you can't seem to stay healthy for longer than a few weeks at a time. Perhaps you are constantly visiting the doctor with colds or random illnesses.

There are any number of issues that are all related to the health of the immune system, the gut, and also the endocrine system which regulates hormones. Hormones are responsible for a whole host of health related issues in the body. Your endocrine system (aka hormone production) is responsible for your reproductive system and how well you are able to procreate, your sleep and wake patterns and your ability to get good sleep, your metabolism and how well your body is able to digest foods and metabolize them so you do not gain weight, and your emotions and how well you are able to adapt to stress and mood swings. These are just a few areas affected by your hormones.

ESSENTIAL OIL MAKE & TAKES *by Jen O'Sullivan*

Your immune system affects practically every area of your body, such as how well your body responds to physical stress and inflammation, how well you are able to ward off disease and sickness, and how your body, along with your gut, controls potential autoimmune disorders and autism. Synthetics are a real threat. Synthetics disrupt your immune and endocrine (hormone) systems. When you remove the synthetics from your life, YOUR LIFE WILL RADICALLY IMPROVE!

Are you ready to swap out your synthetic products with ones using plant-based natural ingredients you make yourself? This book is dedicated to you! Enjoy it, mark it up, make it your go-to recipe book for all things Make & Take!

ESSENTIAL OIL MAKE & TAKES by Jen O'Sullivan

BABY BOTTOM PASTE

Ingredients:
- 4 ounce Glass Jar
- 4 tablespoons Shea Butter
- 2 tablespoons Zinc Oxide powder
- 1 tablespoon Jojoba oil
- 2 tablespoons Aloe Vera gel
- 10 drops of Gentle Baby®
- Starter kit: 5 drops each Lavender and Frankincense

DIY Directions: In a double boiler, melt Shea butter until just melted. Turn off burner and add Jojoba oil, Aloe Vera gel, and essential oils and blend well. Slowly stir in Zinc Oxide powder, a small amount at a time, until it is fully blended. Pour lotion into jar and seal tightly to let cool.

> *Note: Zinc Oxide powder is very fine. Wear gloves and do not allow any to get into your lungs. Do not have small children in the room when working with the powder form of Zinc Oxide. While Zinc Oxide is a natural ingredient and is non-toxic, it should not be inhaled.*

Directions for Use: Apply to baby's bottom as needed during a diaper change.

Party Type: Make & Take 102

BABY GUM SOOTHING SERUM

Ingredients:
- 5ml Dropper Bottle
- Jojoba oil
- 5 drops each Clove and Lavender essential oils
- Starter kit: 5 drops each Lavender and Thieves®

DIY Directions: Combine essential oils in the dropper bottle and swirl to blend. Top off with Jojoba carrier oil.

Directions for Use: Apply to baby's gums as needed.

Party Type: Make & Take 101

ESSENTIAL OIL MAKE & TAKES by Jen O'Sullivan

BABY SCALP SCRUB & SERUM

Ingredients for *Scalp Scrub*:
- 2 ounce Glass Jar
- 2 tablespoons Jojoba oil
- 1 tablespoon Coconut oil (Alternative: Jojoba oil)
- 1-2 tablespoons Baking Soda
- 5 drops Gentle Baby®
- Starter kit: 3 drops each Lavender and Frankincense

DIY Directions: Combine all ingredients and blend well.

Ingredients for *Scalp Serum*:
- 15ml Dropper Bottle
- 1 tablespoon Jojoba oil
- 3 drops each Lavender and Frankincense

DIY Directions: Combine essential oils in the dropper bottle and swirl to blend. Top off with Jojoba oil and swirl to blend.

Directions for Use: Apply *Scalp Scrub* to baby's scalp 2 times daily in a circular motion. Use a warm microfiber cloth to gently rinse off. Apply 2-3 drops of the *Scalp Serum* directly after rubbing off scrub.

Party Type: Make & Take 102

BATH SALTS

Ingredients:
- 8 ounce Mason Jar
- ¾ cup Epsom Salt
- 1 tablespoon Baking Soda
- 8-10 drops of Lavender or blend of choice

DIY Directions: Combine salt and Baking Soda in jar, add essential oil, place lid on tightly, and shake to disperse.

Directions for Use: Pour entire contents into a warm bath and enjoy!

Party Type: Make & Take 101

ESSENTIAL OIL MAKE & TAKES *by Jen O'Sullivan*

BATH SOAK (OATMEAL)

Ingredients:
- 8 ounce Glass Jar
- ½ cup Epsom Salt
- ½ cup Gluten Free Oats (Quick Oats)
- 1 tablespoon Baking Soda
- 15 drops Peace & Calming®
- Starter kit essential oils: Lavender or Stress Away™

DIY Directions: Grind Oats and Epsom Salt in a coffee grinder until it is a fine texture. Add Baking Soda and essential oils. Blend well and place into glass jar.

Directions for Use: Pour 1 cup into a hot bath and soak for 30 minutes.

Party Type: Make & Take 101

BIKINI LINE SERUM

Ingredients:
- 15ml Dropper Bottle
- Grapeseed oil
- 30 drops Grapefruit
- Starter kit essential oils: Lemon

DIY Directions: Combine all ingredients. Fasten on the cap, then swirl the bottle to blend well.

Directions for Use: Apply a dime-size amount over shaved areas right after you towel off from the shower.
NOTE: do not use this if you are going to sun bathe!

Party Type: Make & Take 101

ESSENTIAL OIL MAKE & TAKES by Jen O'Sullivan

BODY SUGAR SCRUB

Ingredients:
- 4 ounce Glass Jar
- ¼ cup Brown Sugar
- ¼ cup Raw Cane Sugar
- 2 tablespoons Grapeseed oil
- 2 tablespoons Organic Honey (optional)
- Melted Raw Coconut oil to desired consistency (Alternative: Grapeseed or Jojoba oil)
- 10-15 drops Lemon

DIY Directions: Combine all ingredients in a bowl and blend to a wet sand consistency. It should not be crumbly, but more soupy in texture. Scoop into jar and place lid on tightly. Do not fill to the top or the oils will seep out.

Directions for Use: Scoop out a handful and scrub over freshly-washed body in the shower. Rinse off with warm water and towel dry for supple soft skin!

Party Type: Make & Take 101

ESSENTIAL OIL MAKE & TAKES *by Jen O'Sullivan*

BODY WASH

Ingredients:
- 8 ounce Glass Bottle or Foaming Soap Dispenser
- ½ cup Liquid Castile Soap
- 4 tablespoons Vegetable Glycerin
- 3 tablespoons Sweet Almond Oil
- 10 drops each Peppermint, Lavender, and Lemon

DIY Directions: Combine all essential oils in bottle and swirl to blend. Add Vegetable Glycerin and Sweet Almond oil and swirl to blend. Add Castile soap and shake well to fully blend.
> *Note: Alternative for use as a Foaming Body Wash: fill foaming soap container to ¼ full. Top off with distilled water and shake to blend.*

Directions for Use: Use in the shower with a loofah or washcloth.

Party Type: Make & Take 101

BUBBLE BATH

Ingredients:
- 4 ounce Glass Bottle
- ½ cup Liquid Castile Soap (Natural Way Organics)
- ¼ cup Vegetable Glycerin
- 2 tablespoons White Granulated Sugar
- 1 Egg White (optional for larger bubbles)
- 10 drops Tangerine
- Starter kit essential oils: Lavender or Citrus Fresh™

DIY Directions: Combine all ingredients and shake to blend.

Directions for Use: Pour half of contents under running bath water. Place remaining contents in refrigerator to be used within a week.
> *Note: Natural bubble bath recipes generally do not work. I have tried too many to count and all have failed. This is the best one I have come up with. The trick is using the correct type of Castile soap. You need to use one that is made out of Saponified Coconut oil. Natural Way Organics is a good one. The bubbles will not compare to store-bought bubble bath but you will have fun for a minute or two and won't have to deal with all the nasty chemicals in the store-bought ones.*

Party Type: Make & Take 102

ESSENTIAL OIL MAKE & TAKES by Jen O'Sullivan

CAR VENT DIFFUSER

Ingredients:
- 1 Clothespin
- Wood Glue
- Raw Wood or Cork Embellishments
- 5 drops Peppermint or blend of choice

DIY Directions: Glue on embellishments to your liking. Allow to fully dry.

Directions for Use: Apply essential oil to cork or raw wood and click clothespin onto air vent. Run air as normal based on desired temperature. This can also work well for hotel rooms. Clip onto air conditioner outflow vent and run air to freshen the room.

Party Type: Make & Take 101

ESSENTIAL OIL MAKE & TAKES *by Jen O'Sullivan*

COOL-DOWN SPRAY

Ingredients:
- 2 ounce Glass Spray Bottle
- 1 ounce Distilled Water
- 1 ounce Witch Hazel
- 20 drops Peppermint

DIY Directions: Combine the essential oil and Witch Hazel in the bottle and swirl to blend. Top off with distilled water and swirl to blend.

Directions for Use: Spray liberally on skin to cool down as needed. For men, this works great to spray across the shoulders and back. For women, during menopause, spray anywhere as needed. Do not spray in eyes. If you want to spray on the face, sight down, close eyes tightly, mist over face, and keep eyes closed until mist dries completely.

Party Type: Make & Take 101

CRITTER SPRAY

Ingredients:
- 2 ounce Spray Bottle
- Distilled Water
- Witch Hazel
- 1 tablespoon Jojoba oil
- 100 drops (yes, 100 drops) Purification®
- Starter kit essential oils: no alternative

DIY Directions: Combine the essential oil and Jojoba oil in the dropper bottle and swirl to blend. Add Witch Hazel to half full and swirl to blend. Top off with distilled water and swirl again.

Directions for Use: Spray liberally on exposed skin every 1-2 hours when outdoors.

Party Type: Make & Take 102

Essential oil MAKE & TAKES *by Jen O'Sullivan*

FACE CLEANSER

Ingredients:
- 2-4 ounce Glass Jar
- Organic Raw Coconut Oil (Alternative: Sweet Almond Oil)
- 5 drops each Lavender and Frankincense

DIY Directions: Melt Coconut oil in a double boiler until just melted. Remove from heat immediately. Pour melted Coconut oil into glass jar. Add essential oils and swirl jar to blend. Place in refrigerator to set.

Directions for Use: Use a warm facecloth over your face for 15 seconds. Allow warm cloth to open pores. Scoop out about a tablespoon of Face Cleanser and rub all over face and eye area. Massage in to fully remove all makeup. Wipe off makeup with tissue or cotton pads. Discard and continue to wipe with clean tissue until makeup is fully off. Take the washcloth and run under warm water. Apply over face to finish for a spa-like experience.

Party Type: Make & Take 101

Azuki Beans

FACE EXFOLIATOR

Ingredients:
- 4 ounce Glass Jar
- Organic Raw Coconut oil (Alternative: Sweet Almond oil)
- ¼ cup Azuki Beans (dried and ground in a coffee grinder)
- Alternatives: Ground Almonds, Baking Soda, or Cane Sugar
- Distilled Water
- 20 drops Lemon and 10 drops Tea Tree
- Starter kit essential oils: 10 drops each Lemon, Lavender, and Frankincense

DIY Directions: Melt Coconut oil in a double boiler until just melted. Remove from heat immediately. Pour melted Coconut oil into glass bowl. Add essential oils and ground Azuki beans and blend well. Add some water to desired consistency. Scoop into jar.

Directions for Use: After face is fully cleansed, use a warm facecloth over your face for 15 seconds. Apply a small amount of Face Exfoliator in small circular motions. Rinse with warm water, then use a final rinse/splash of cool water to close up pores.

Party Type: Make & Take 102

ESSENTIAL OIL MAKE & TAKES *by Jen O'Sullivan*

EYE SERUM

Ingredients:
- 5ml Dropper Bottle
- Organic Raw Rosehip Seed and Jamaican Black Castor Oil
- 5 drops each Gentle Baby™, Frankincense, and Myrrh, 3 drops each Sandalwood (optional) and Patchouli, 1 drop Rose (optional)
- Starter kit essential oils: 5 drops each Lavender and Frankincense, and 3 drops Lemon

DIY Directions: Combine all essential oils in the dropper bottle. Swirl to blend. Add Jamaican Black Castor oil to about ½ full and fill to ¾ full with Rosehip Seed oil, leaving room for the dropper. Fasten the dropper cap on, then swirl the bottle to blend well.

Directions for Use: Apply 2-4 drops around eyes before bed. Gently pat around eyes. Do not get any directly into eyes. Not for use during the day if going into sunlight.

Party Type: Make & Take 102

FACE SERUM (ALL SKIN TYPES)

Ingredients:
- 10ml Dropper Bottle
- Organic Raw Grapeseed oil
- 8-10 drops each of Lavender and Frankincense

DIY Directions: Combine Lavender and Frankincense in the dropper bottle. Swirl to blend the two oils. Add Grapeseed oil to about ¾ full, leaving room for the dropper. Fasten the dropper cap on, then swirl the bottle to blend well. This one is a customer favorite!

Directions for Use: Apply a dime-size amount (about 8 drops) all over freshly-washed face, neck, and back of hands both morning and night.

Party Type: Make & Take 101

Frankincense Resin

FACE SERUM (BLEMISH SUPPORT)
Ingredients:
- 10ml Dropper Bottle
- Organic Raw Grapeseed oil or Pumpkin Seed oil
- 10 drops Tea Tree, and 5 drops Valor®
- Starter kit essential oils: 5 drops each Lavender, Lemon, and Frankincense, plus 2 drops Valor®

DIY Directions: Add essential oils and swirl to blend. Fil with Grapeseed or Pumpkin Seed oil to about ¾ full, leaving room for the dropper. Fasten the cap on, then swirl the bottle to blend well.

Directions for Use: Apply a dime-size amount (about 8 drops) all over freshly-washed face, neck, or anywhere that is needed, morning and night.

Party Type: Make & Take 101

FACE TONER SPRAY
Ingredients:
- 4 ounce Glass Spray Bottle
- 4 ounces Distilled Water
- 5 drops each Lavender, Sacred Frankincense, and Sandalwood
- Starter kit essential oils: 5 drops each Lavender and Frankincense

DIY Directions: Combine all essential oils into spray bottle and swirl around to blend. Add distilled water or hydrosol and shake to mix.

Directions for Use: Spray directly onto face morning and night or anytime as needed. Keep in the refrigerator for longer shelf-life. Use product within 1-2 weeks if not in the refrigerator, or up to 1 month if kept in the refrigerator.

Party Type: Make & Take 102

ESSENTIAL OIL MAKE & TAKES *by Jen O'Sullivan*

FINGERNAIL SUPPORT

Ingredients:
- 5ml Dropper Bottle
- Jojoba oil
- 5 drops each Lemon, Lavender, Frankincense, and Myrrh (optional)

DIY Directions: Combine the essential oils in the dropper bottle and swirl to blend. Add Jojoba oil and swirl to blend.

Directions for Use: Massage onto fingernails twice a day.

Party Type: Make & Take 101 or 102

FIZZIES (BATH BOMBS)

Ingredients:
- Glass Jar
- Flexible Mold
- 1 cup Citric Acid
- 1 cup Baking Soda
- 1 ½ cups Corn Starch
- 1-2 teaspoons Grapeseed Oil
- Plant Based Food Coloring
- 1-3 drops Lavender or calming essential oil

DIY Directions: Combine Citric Acid, Baking Soda, and Corn Starch. Slowly drizzle a small amount of Grapeseed oil into the mix, kneading until it feels like wet sand. Be careful not to add too much Grapeseed oil otherwise you may activate the Citric Acid and ruin the mix. Add a natural, plant-based coloring. Smooth into a flexible mold of your choice or plastic globe molds. Add 1-3 drops Lavender essential oil per mold depending on mold size. Let dry completely. Gently pop Fizzies out of molds and store in an airtight glass jar.

Directions for Use: Drop 1-2 Fizzies into your warm bath.

Party Type: Make & Take 102

~ 18 ~

ESSENTIAL OIL MAKE & TAKES by Jen O'Sullivan

FRAGRANCE

Ingredients:
- 5ml Fragrance Atomizer
- Witch Hazel
- Essential oil Blend of Choice
    - *Create one of the following recipes:*
        - ORANGE 50/50 BAR: 8 drops Tangerine essential oil and 2 drops Vanilla Absolute (Not Grocery Store Extract)
        - FRESH & CLEAN: 3 drops each Copaiba, Lavender, Lemon, and Peppermint
        - LIME CAKE: 3 drops each Lavender and Cedarwood, plus 6 drops Lime and 2-4 drops Vanilla Absolute.
        - Starter kit essential oil: 8 drops Stress Away™

DIY Directions: Combine the essential oils in the atomizer and swirl to blend. Add Witch Hazel and shake to mix well.

Directions for Use: Spray on pulse points as desired.

ESSENTIAL OIL MAKE & TAKES by Jen O'Sullivan

HAND LOTION

Ingredients:
- 4 ounce Glass Jar
- ¼ cup Shea Butter
- 2 tablespoons Sweet Almond oil
- 1 tablespoon Beeswax (Vegan Alternative: Candelilla Wax)
- 20 drops Lime, 10 drops each Lavender, Cedarwood, and Copaiba
- Starter kit essential oils: 10 drops each Lemon, Lavender, and Frankincense
- *NOTE: the citrus oils help brighten and even tone on the hands. If you go into the sun often, omit the citrus oils.*

DIY Directions: Combine essential oils in a small bowl and swirl to blend well. Add Sweet Almond oil and swirl again to blend well. Set to the side. Melt beeswax in a double boiler, add Shea Butter and melt together with beeswax, stirring constantly. Remove from heat. Add Sweet Almond/essential oil blend to the mix and stir well. Pour into glass jar and cool in the refrigerator to set.

Directions for Use: Apply to hands as needed.

Party Type:
Make & Take 102

ESSENTIAL OIL MAKE & TAKES *by Jen O'Sullivan*

HAND SOAP (FOAMING)

Ingredients:
- 8 ounce Foaming Hand Soap Dispenser
- 6 ounces Distilled Water
- 2 tablespoons Liquid Castile Soap
- ¼ tablespoon Organic Sweet Almond oil
- 10 drops Thieves®, Lavender, or Citrus Fresh™

DIY Directions: Combine all ingredients into dispenser making sure to leave extra room for the pump.

Directions for Use: Pump some foam, and wash those hands!

Party Type: Make & Take 101

HAND SCRUBBING BALLS

Ingredients:
- Glass Jar
- Mini Globe Molds
- 1 cup Epsom Salt
- 1 cup Baking Soda
- ¼ cup Water
- 10-20 drops Lavender

DIY Directions: Grind Epsom Salt in a coffee grinder until it becomes a fine powder. Blend together with Baking Soda. Add 10-20 drops essential oil, then slowly mix in water until it becomes a stiff cookie dough consistency. Roll into small balls and place on wax paper or place into molds. Make balls about ¾ the size of the mold as the mix will expand as it dries. If using a mold, tape it shut or use a weight to keep it closed while it dries. Once fully dry, put balls into a glass container next to the sink.

Directions for Use: Use one ball to give your hands a good clean scrub.

Party Type: Make & Take 102

ESSENTIAL OIL MAKE & TAKES by Jen O'Sullivan

HAIR CONDITIONING RINSE

Ingredients:
- Large Glass Water Jug
- 1 cup Apple Cider Vinegar
- 1 cup Distilled Water
- 1 tablespoon Organic Honey (optional)
- 10 drops each Peppermint and Lavender, and 5 drops Rosemary (optional)

DIY Directions: Combine all essential oils into glass water jug and swirl to blend. Add honey and swirl to blend. Pour in Apple Cider Vinegar and swirl to blend again. Add distilled water and blend well.

Directions for Use: Apply to freshly-washed, damp hair and massage for 2 minutes. Rinse out completely, towel dry, and apply Hair Serum to the ends of hair. Style as usual.

Party Type: Make & Take 102

HAIR DEEP CLEANSER

Ingredients:
- 2 ounce Dropper Bottle
- 1.75 ounces Distilled Water
- 20 drops each Tea Tree, Lemon, and Rosemary
- Starter kit Essential oils: 20 drops each Lemon and Lavender, 10 drops Frankincense

DIY Directions: Combine all essential oils into dropper bottle and swirl to blend. Top off with distilled water and shake to mix.

Directions for Use: Place dropper bottle into a bowl of hot water to warm up for 2 minutes. Wet hair in a warm shower. Apply directly to scalp while mix is still warm and rub into scalp and hair. Leave on for a minimum of 2 minutes while in the shower or a maximum of 10 minutes with a shower cap on. Rinse well and apply conditioner of choice.

Party Type: Make & Take 102

ESSENTIAL OIL MAKE & TAKES by Jen O'Sullivan

HAIR DEEP CONDITIONER

Ingredients:
- 1 Ripe Avocado
- 2 tablespoons Organic Honey
- 1 tablespoon Jamaican Black Castor Oil
- 5 drops each Geranium, Lavender, and Sandalwood
- Starter kit Essential oils: 5 drops each Lavender, Peppermint, and Frankincense

DIY Directions: Combine all essential oils into bowl and swirl around to blend. Mash avocado until completely smooth and creamy. Use blender if necessary. Add Jamaican Black Castor oil and continue to blend. Add essential oil blend and mix well. Use recipe right after you make it. This is for a single use.

Directions for Use: Apply the entire mix to damp hair and cover with a plastic cap. Leave on for 30-60 minutes. Rinse completely out and apply Hair Serum to the ends of hair. Style as usual.

Party Type: Make & Take 102

ESSENTIAL OIL MAKE & TAKES *by Jen O'Sullivan*

HAIR DETANGLING SPRAY

Ingredients:
- 4 ounce Glass Spray Bottle
- 2 ounces Distilled Water or Lavender Hydrosol
- 1 ½ teaspoons Apple Cider Vinegar
- 10 drops each Rosemary, Lavender, and Cedarwood
- Starter kit essential oils: 10 drops each Lavender and Peppermint or Stress Away™

DIY Directions: Combine all essential oils into the glass spray bottle and swirl to blend. (Optional: Wait 24 hours to allow oils to fully synergize.) Add 1.5 teaspoons of Apple Cider Vinegar. Shake bottle to fully blend ingredients. Add 2 ounces distilled water or Lavender hydrosol and shake again.

Directions for Use: Spray on dry or damp hair as needed. Shake gently before each use. Use entire spray within 2 weeks to maintain freshness of oils. Discard any unused portion after two weeks as oils may oxidize.

Party Type: Make & Take 102

HAIR DETANGLING SPRAY (EASY VERSION)

Ingredients:
- 4 ounce Glass Spray Bottle
- 3.5 ounces Distilled Water
- 1 tablespoon Copaiba Vanilla Conditioner™

DIY Directions: Pour distilled water into glass spray bottle, add Copaiba Vanilla Conditioner™ and shake well.

Directions for Use: Spray on dry or damp hair as needed. Shake gently before each use. For added scent, consider adding 5 drops of Lavender essential oil.

Party Type: Make & Take 101

Essential oil MAKE & TAKES by Jen O'Sullivan

Cocoa Beans & Powder

HAIR DRY SHAMPOO

Ingredients:
- Empty Spice Shaker
- ¼ cup Cornstarch (Alternative: Arrowroot)
- 1 tablespoon Baking Soda
- Optional for dark hair: 2 tablespoons Cocoa Powder
- 6 drops Lime, plus 3 drops each Tea Tree, Rosemary, Lavender, and Cedarwood
- Starter kit essential oils: 6 drops Lemon, plus 3 drops each Lavender and Peppermint

DIY Directions: Combine all essential oils into a clean bottle and swirl around to blend. Combine all dry ingredients into shaker container and shake to mix. Add essential oil blend and shake to mix.

Directions for Use: Sprinkle dry shampoo onto the roots of your hair and massage into your scalp. Leave on for 2 minutes, then shake out and brush through. To add shine back on ends, use Hair Serum.

Party Type: Make & Take 102

ESSENTIAL OIL MAKE & TAKES *by Jen O'Sullivan*

HAIR FOLLICLE SPRAY

Ingredients:
- 4 ounce Glass Spray Bottle
- 3 ounces Distilled Water or Homemade Hydrosol using Lavender, Peppermint, or Rosemary (See Hydrosol recipe)
- **FOR WOMEN:** 20 drops each Peppermint, Lavender, Cedarwood, Rosemary, Cypress, Thyme, and Clary Sage essential oils
- **FOR MEN:** 20 drops each Peppermint, Lavender, Cedarwood, Rosemary, Cypress, Thyme, and Northern Lights Black Spruce™
- Starter kit essential oils: 20 drops each Peppermint, Lavender, and Frankincense

DIY Directions: Combine all essential oils into spray bottle and swirl to blend. Add distilled water or hydrosol and shake to mix.

Directions for Use: Spray directly onto scalp morning and night. Keep in the refrigerator for longer shelf life. Use product within 1-2 weeks if not in the refrigerator, or up to one month if kept in the refrigerator.

Party Type: Make & Take 102

Peppermint Leaves

ESSENTIAL OIL MAKE & TAKES *by Jen O'Sullivan*

HAIR SERUM (SMOOTHER)

Ingredients:
- 15ml Dropper Bottle
- Jojoba Oil or Grapeseed oil
- 40 drops Jamaican Black Castor oil
- 10 drops each Frankincense, Tea Tree, Rosemary, Lavender, Cedarwood, Clary Sage, and Lemon
- Starter kit essential oils: 10 drops each Frankincense, Lavender, Lemon, and Peppermint (or try Stress Away™ alone)

DIY Directions: Combine all essential oils into a 15ml bottle and swirl to blend. Add 40 drops of Jamaican Black Castor oil and top off with Jojoba oil for coarse or wavy/curly hair or Grapeseed oil for straight or fine hair. Swirl bottle to blend.

Directions for Use: Use 2-5 drops. Rub hands together to warm up the oil and apply to the ends of hair first, working your way up to mid-shaft. Do not apply to roots or top of head. Use the small leftovers to gently pat down flyaway hairs.

Party Type: Make & Take 102

HAIR SHAMPOO

Ingredients:
- 8-16 ounce Hard Plastic or Glass Pump Bottle
- Distilled Water
- Castile Soap
- 20 drops Lavender and 10 drops Peppermint (or blend of choice)

DIY Directions: Combine essential oils into pump bottle and swirl to blend. Fill halfway with Castile soap and swirl to blend. Top off with distilled water and shake to mix.

Directions for Use: Pump a generous amount into hands and lather onto wet hair. Rinse and repeat if desired.

> *Note: If you have been using traditional shampoo, expect a transition period of up to 6 months while your hair and scalp adjust. During this period, it is important to use Hair Follicle Spray and Hair Serum on wash days, and as needed on in-between days. You can use Copaiba Vanilla Shampoo™ to help with the transition period.*

Party Type: Make & Take 102

ESSENTIAL OIL MAKE & TAKES by Jen O'Sullivan

HAIR SPLIT END SPRAY

Ingredients:
- 2-4 ounce Glass Spray Bottle
- 2 ounces Distilled Water or Lavender Hydrosol
- 1 teaspoon Jojoba oil
- 10 drops each Frankincense, Rosemary, Lavender, Cedarwood, and Clary Sage
- Starter kit essential oils: 10 drops each Frankincense and Lavender

DIY Directions: Combine all essential oils into the glass spray bottle and swirl to blend. Add 1 teaspoon of Jojoba oil. Shake bottle to fully blend ingredients. Add 2 ounces distilled water and shake again.

Directions for Use: Spray on dry or damp hair as needed 1-2 times per day. Shake gently before each use. Use entire spray within 2 weeks to maintain freshness of oils. Discard any unused portion after two weeks as oils may oxidize.

Party Type: Make & Take 102

HAIR SHINE SPRAY

Ingredients:
- 2 ounce Glass Spray Bottle
- 2 ounces Distilled Water or Lavender Hydrosol
- 10 drops each Sandalwood, Rosemary, Copaiba, and Lavender
- Starter kit essential oils: 10 drops each Lavender

DIY Directions: Combine all essential oils into the glass spray bottle and swirl to blend. Add 2 ounces distilled water and shake to fully blend ingredients.

Directions for Use: Spray on dry or damp hair as needed 1-2 times per day. Shake gently before each use. Use entire spray within 2 weeks to maintain freshness of oils. Discard any unused portion after two weeks as oils may oxidize.

Party Type: Make & Take 102

ESSENTIAL OIL MAKE & TAKES by Jen O'Sullivan

HEEL AND FOOT CREAM

Ingredients:
- 4 ounce Glass Jar
- ¼ cup Shea Butter
- ¼ cup Raw Coconut oil
- 2 tablespoons Beeswax (Vegan Alternative: Candelilla Wax)
- 10 drops Frankincense, 10 drops Lavender, 10 drops Bergamot, 5 drops Tea Tree, and 5 drops Oregano essential oils
- Starter kit essential oils: 10 drops each Frankincense, Lavender, Lemon, and Peppermint

DIY Directions: Combine the essential oils in the glass jar and swirl to blend. Place the lid on and set to the side. Melt Beeswax in a double boiler, add Shea Butter and melt together, stirring constantly. Remove from heat and add Coconut oil and mix well. While still liquid, pour contents into glass jar containing the essential oils. Place lid on tightly and shake to blend well. Place in refrigerator to set.

Directions for Use: Massage onto feet morning and night.

Party Type: Make & Take 102

Shea Nuts & Butter

ESSENTIAL OIL MAKE & TAKES by Jen O'Sullivan

HOME: CANDLES (LAVENDER BUD)

Ingredients:
- 1-2 sheets Natural Beeswax (8" x 16" Natural Color)
- 1-2 feet Candle Wick
- 2 tablespoons Organic Lavender Buds
- 5-10 drops Lavender

DIY Directions: Working on a flat, clean surface, place one sheet of beeswax in front of you. Measure the short width of the sheet and cut candle wick to ½ inch longer than the short width. In a separate small bowl, wind up cut candle wick and drip 5-10 drops of Lavender essential oil to fully saturate the wick. Pull wick out and pour Lavender buds into bowl. Unwind wick and place straight along the very end of the short end of the beeswax sheet, leaving ½ inch of wick sticking over one end (this will be the top of your candle). Starting from one corner, fold over a very small part of the beeswax to wrap around the wick. Use a hairdryer to warm up the wax a bit to make it more pliable. Do not melt. Continue working up the wick, wrapping it with the edge of the beeswax. Once the entire wick is wrapped, start to roll the wick up in the beeswax like you would roll up a carpet. Keep the roll as tight as possible without smashing down the hexagon pattern too much. When there are 4 inches left on the roll, stop rolling and sprinkle Lavender Buds on the inside of the leftover 4 inches. Spread out evenly or make a pattern, making sure they are all flat on the beeswax while keeping the final ¼ inch edge free and clear. Gently pat them down. Continue to roll the candle. Once finished, smooth the final ¼ inch edge down using the warmth of your fingers to tack it down. Using glue, apply Lavender Buds to the outside bottom for decoration. Trim wick to ¼ inch. Tap down base edge to stand up.

Directions for Use: Create two candles and wrap with ribbon for a wonderful gift. Use as decoration in a bathroom, or light for a peaceful Lavender Candle experience. Remember to use a candle base to catch any wax drips.

Party Type: Make & Take 101 or 102

ESSENTIAL OIL MAKE & TAKES *by Jen O'Sullivan*

HOME: DEGREASER
Ingredients:
- Large Hard Plastic or Glass Spray Bottle
- 2 cups Distilled Water
- 1 cup White Vinegar
- 1 tablespoon Baking Soda
- 1 teaspoon Castile Soap
- 20 drops each Orange and Lemon
- Starter kit essential oils: 20 drops Thieves® and 20 drops Lemon

DIY Directions: Combine all ingredients and shake to blend.

Directions for Use: Shake before each use. Spray liberally on surface and let sit for 5 minutes. Spray again to keep wet for a total of 15 minutes. Wipe clean.

Party Type: Make & Take 102

HOME: DRAWER SACHETS (LAVENDER)
Ingredients:
- 2 Quilting Squares (Zig-Zag Edged)
- Fabric Glue
- Small Funnel
- 2 tablespoons Organic Lavender Buds
- 5 drops Lavender and Cedarwood (optional)

DIY Directions: Place one quilting square with the outside facing down. Edge with fabric glue about 1/8 inch from the edge all the way around, leaving a 1 inch area unglued on one side. The glue will look like a boxy letter "C". Place second quilting square directly on top with outside facing up. Let fully dry. Place Lavender buds in a small bowl and infuse with Lavender and Cedarwood essential oils. Cover and shake to mix. Once quilting squares are fully dry, slide a funnel into the small opening on the side and fill with Lavender buds. Glue the opening shut and place a weight on it to keep tacked down. Once fully dry, shake sachet to activate the scent.

Directions for Use: Place Lavender Sachet into lingerie drawer or small space, such as a car or office drawer.

Party Type: Make & Take 101

ESSENTIAL OIL MAKE & TAKES *by Jen O'Sullivan*

HOME: ROOM FRESHENER

Ingredients:
- 4 ounce Glass Spray Bottle
- 2 ounces Distilled Water
- 2 ounces Witch Hazel
- 8-10 drops of essential oil of choice

DIY Directions: Fill bottle with distilled water and Witch Hazel, then add essential oils and shake to blend. For a kid's room spritzer, use Stress Away™ for bedtime calming and decorate with a fun label for "Monster-Away Spray."

Directions for Use: Spray in the air as needed or directly onto pillows and fabric.

Party Type: Make & Take 101

HOME: WINDOW CLEANER

Ingredients:
- Large Hard Plastic or Glass Spray Bottle
- 2 cups Distilled Water
- ¼ cup White Vinegar
- ¼ cup Rubbing Alcohol
- 1 tablespoon Cornstarch
- 2 ounces Witch Hazel
- 10 drops of Thieves® and 10 drops Orange or Lemon

DIY Directions: Combine all ingredients into spray bottle and shake to blend.

Directions for Use: Shake well before each use. Spray on glass and surfaces for a streak-free shine. Use a microfiber cloth so there is no lint left on the windows.

Party Type: Make & Take 102

ESSENTIAL OIL MAKE & TAKES by Jen O'Sullivan

HYDROSOL

Ingredients:
- Fresh Organic Plants such as Peppermint, Lavender, or Rosemary. Make sure they are the correct Latin binomial. *Mentha piperita, Lavandula angustifolia, or Rosmarinus officinalis.*
- Large Stainless Steel Pot with Lid
- Small Ramekin
- Medium Bowl to fit on top of Ramekin inside the large pot
- Distilled Water
- Ice Cubes
- 2-4 ounce Glass Spray Bottle
- Suggested essential oils to add: Lavender, Peppermint, Frankincense, or blend of choice

DIY Directions: Place ramekin upside down in large pot. Place medium bowl on top. There should be at least two inches of space around the entire pot area from the medium bowl outside edge to the large pot outside edge. Add cut up plants in the large pot at the bottom around the ramekin. Fill with distilled water to just cover the plants. Put on low heat. Do not allow water to boil. It should be hot enough to have steam but not boil. Place the large pot lid over the pot upside down so the lid handle is underneath. Place ice on the upside-down lid. As the steam rises, the ice will cool it causing it to create liquid condensation that will then drip down into the medium size bowl. This is the Hydrosol. Allow the water to collect for 20-30 minutes. Continue to add ice as needed to the upside-down lid. Pour Hydrosol into 4 ounce bottle and store in the refrigerator.

Directions for Use:
Add your favorite essential oils to your Hydrosol and label for use. Common uses are for hair and face sprays. Store in refrigerator for longer shelf life.

Party Type:
Make & Take 102

Lavender Flowers

ESSENTIAL OIL MAKE & TAKES *by Jen O'Sullivan*

LIP BALM

Makes: About 1 Dozen Tubes

Ingredients:
- 2 tablespoons Shea Butter
- 2 tablespoons Raw Coconut oil (Alternative: Jojoba oil)
- 1 ½ tablespoons Beeswax Pellets. Use 2 Tbsp. for stiffer lip balm. (Vegan Alternative: Candelilla Wax)
- 30 drops essential oil (suggestions: Peppermint, Lavender, Grapefruit, or your favorite blend)

DIY Directions: On wax paper, line up tubes about 3 inches apart with caps off on a clear surface. Melt Shea Butter, Coconut oil, and Beeswax together in a double boiler. Stir constantly until fully melted. Turn off burner and add essential oils. Blend in well. While still warm and melted, use a pipette to fill lip balm tubes. Let tubes cool completely at room temperature before placing caps on.

Directions for Use: Apply to lips as needed!

Party Type: Make & Take 102

LIP SCRUB

Makes: About 6 Mini Containers

Ingredients:
- 3 teaspoons Brown Sugar
- 2 tablespoons Raw Coconut oil (Alternative: Jojoba oil)
- 1 teaspoon Molasses (Alternative: Organic Honey)
- 3 drops Lemon, 2 drops Ginger, 1 drop Nutmeg, 1 drop Cinnamon Bark
- Starter kit Essential oils: 3 drops Lemon, 2 drops Thieves®

DIY Directions: Blend all essential oils in small clean bottle and swirl to blend. Set aside. In small bowl, blend Coconut oil, Brown Sugar, and Molasses until mixed well. Add essential oil blend. Scoop into mini jars.

Directions for Use: Apply small amount to lips and gently scrub in a circular motion. Wipe off excess to reveal smooth, soft lips.

Party Type: Make & Take 101

ESSENTIAL OIL MAKE & TAKES by Jen O'Sullivan

MAKEUP REMOVING PADS
Ingredients:
- 4 ounce Glass Jar (to fit cotton rounds)
- 24 Cotton Rounds
- ¼ cup Witch Hazel
- 2 tablespoons Sweet Almond oil
- 2 tablespoons Distilled Water
- 2 teaspoons Castile Soap
- 5 drops each of Lavender and Frankincense

DIY Directions: Stack cotton rounds into the glass jar and set to the side. In a separate mixing bowl, add essential oils and swirl to blend. Add Sweet Almond oil and Castile soap and swirl to blend. Add both Witch Hazel and Distilled Water and blend well. Pour mix over the cotton rounds in the glass jar.

Directions for Use: Remove makeup with pads.

Party Type: Make & Take 101

LUCY LIBIDO'S "SKINAMINT"
(EDIBLE PERSONAL LUBRICANT) www.lucylibido.com

Ingredients:
- ½ teaspoon Beeswax
- 3 teaspoons Raw Coconut oil
- 3 teaspoons Edible Grapeseed oil
- ¼ - ½ teaspoon Agave
- 4-5 drops Peppermint Vitality™
- 8 drops Grapefruit Vitality™
- 2 drops Orange Vitality™

DIY Directions: Melt the Beeswax and Coconut oil together. Remove from heat. Add the Agave and Grapeseed oil. Stir in the essential oils. Store in a pump top bottle or dropper bottle.

Directions for Use: Named by Mr. Libido as tasting like "Skinamint", this edible lube will change the way you think about flavored lubes... no nasty chemical flavor, and it feels AHHH AHHH AHHmaaaazing on. It contains no preservatives, so check for freshness each time it's used.

Party Type: Make & Take 102

ESSENTIAL OIL MAKE & TAKES *by Jen O'Sullivan*

MANLY AFTERSHAVE

Ingredients:
- 15ml Dropper Bottle
- Witch Hazel
- 30 drops Aloe Vera Juice
- 5 drops each Myrrh, Frankincense, and Bergamot, plus 10 drops Northern Lights Black Spruce™
- Starter kit essential oils: 15 drops Thieves® or 5 drops each Frankincense and Peppermint

DIY Directions: Combine essential oils in dropper bottle and swirl to blend. Add Aloe Vera juice and swirl to blend. Top off with Witch Hazel, place dropper cap on tightly, and shake to blend.

Directions for Use: Shake bottle before opening. Apply a small amount into the palm of your hand, rub hands together and pat all over freshly-shaved skin.

Party Type: Make & Take 102

MANLY BEARD BALM

Ingredients:
- 4 ounce Glass Jar
- 3 tablespoons Raw Coconut oil or Sweet Almond oil
- 2 tablespoons Shea Butter or Mango Butter
- 1-2 tablespoon Beeswax (based on desired stiffness, add more to make more stiff, less to make smoother)
- 10 drops Sandalwood, 6 drops Bergamot, 3 drops Clove
- Starter kit essential oils: 10 drops Frankincense, 6 drops Lemon, 3 drops Peppermint

DIY Directions: Cover a low heat double boiler, melt beeswax until just melted. Add Shea or Mango Butter and stir until melted. Add Coconut or Sweet Almond oil and continue to stir. Combine all essential oils into jar and swirl around to blend. Remove from heat and pour into jar with essential oils. Place lid on tightly and swirl to blend. Do not open until fully cooled and set.

Directions for Use: Scoop out a small amount, rub in hands to warm up, and apply to beard as usual. Store in a cool dry place.

Party Type: Make & Take 102

ESSENTIAL OIL MAKE & TAKES by Jen O'Sullivan

MANLY BEARD OIL

Ingredients:
- 10ml Dropper Bottle
- Jojoba Oil
- 9 drops Patchouli, 6 drops Bergamot, 4 drops Clove, 4 drops Rosemary, 3 drops Cedarwood, and 2 drops Lemongrass
- Starter kit essential oils: 10 drops Frankincense and 5 drops Lemon

DIY Directions: Combine essential oils in dropper bottle and swirl to blend. Top off with Jojoba oil and swirl to blend.

Directions for Use: Apply small amount to beard as needed.

Party Type: Make & Take 102

MANLY MUSCLE SUPPORT

Ingredients:
- 10ml Dropper Bottle
- Grapeseed Oil
- 20 drops each PanAway®, Peppermint, and Lavender (add Copaiba for extra support)

DIY Directions: Combine essential oil in dropper bottle and swirl to blend. Top off with Grapeseed oil and swirl to blend.

Directions for Use: Apply to muscles before and after a workout.

Party Type: Make & Take 102

Essential oil MAKE & TAKES by Jen O'Sullivan

Pink Himalayan Sea Salt

MOUTHWASH

Ingredients:
- 8 ounce Glass Jar
- Slightly less than 1 cup Distilled Water
- 2 teaspoons Calcium Carbonate Powder (optional)
- ¼ teaspoon Pink Himalayan Sea Salt
- 10 drops Peppermint, 8 drops Thieves®, and 5 drops Lemon

DIY Directions: Blend all essential oils in small, clean bottle and swirl to blend. Set aside. In 8 ounce jar, add distilled water, Calcium Carbonate, and Pink Himalayan Sea Salt. Shake to mix. Add essential oil blend and shake to mix.

Directions for Use: Gargle morning and night with ½ ounce, then spit out for a fresh clean mouth.

Party Type: Make & Take 102

ESSENTIAL OIL MAKE & TAKES *by Jen O'Sullivan*

NIPPLE BUTTER (FOR NURSING MOMMY)

Ingredients:
- 4 ounce Glass Jar
- 3 tablespoons Raw Coconut Oil (Alternative: Jojoba Oil)
- 2 tablespoons Cocoa Butter
- 1½ tablespoons Beeswax (Alternative: Candelilla Wax)
- 5 drops each Helichrysum, Geranium, Myrrh, Frankincense, and Lavender
- Starter kit essential oils: 10 drops each Frankincense and Lavender

DIY Directions: Combine essential oils in jar and swirl to blend. Melt Beeswax in a double boiler until just melted. Add Cocoa Butter and stir until melted. Turn off burner and add Coconut oil. Continue to stir until fully blended. Pour mix into jar containing essential oils. Place lid on and swirl jar to blend well.

Directions for Use: Apply to nipples as needed between nursing.

Party Type: Make & Take 102

POTTY-POURRI SPRAY

Ingredients:
- 4 ounce Glass Spray Bottle
- ¼ cup Witch Hazel
- 2 tablespoons Everclear® Grain Alcohol (190 Proof Vodka)
- 2 tablespoons Vegetable Glycerin
- 30 drops Thieves® essential oil

DIY Directions: Combine all ingredients in glass spray bottle. Shake vigorously to blend.

Directions for Use: Spray liberally onto toilet bowl water surface prior to use.

Party Type: Make & Take 102

ESSENTIAL OIL MAKE & TAKES by Jen O'Sullivan

ROLLERBALLS

Ingredients:
- 5ml Rollerball
- Organic Raw Grapeseed Oil
- 8-12 drops essential oil recipe of choice

Create one of the following combos:
- Sleep/Focus Support: Stress Away™ or Peace & Calming®
- Chest Rub: Raven™
- Happy Tummy: DiGize™
- Shoulder/Foot Massage: PanAway®
- Courage: 5 drops each Valor®, Frankincense, and Lavender
- Crave Support: 4 drops each Peppermint and Citrus Fresh™
- Holiday Cheer: 5 drops Lemon and 3 drops Thieves®
- Breathe Support: 4 drops each Lavender, Lemon, and Peppermint

DIY Directions: Add essential oils to the 5ml rollerball and top off with Grapeseed oil.

Directions for Use:
- **Sleep/Focus Support Roller:** Apply to the back of the neck, along the spine, on the wrists, or on the big toes.
- **Critter Control Roller:** Apply all over the bottom of the feet and along the hairline.
- **Shoulder/Foot Massage Roller:** Apply over the shoulder area or feet and massage in.
- **Breathe Support Roller:** Apply on the skull behind the ears and down both jaw-lines.

Party Type:
Make & Take 101

Grapeseed Oil

ESSENTIAL OIL MAKE & TAKES *by Jen O'Sullivan*

SCALP SERUM MASK

Ingredients:
- 15ml Dropper Bottle
- Jamaican Black Castor oil
- 10 drops each of any three or five of the following essential oils: Peppermint, Tea Tree, Frankincense, Lavender, Cedarwood, Rosemary, Clary Sage, Thyme, Cypress, Northern Lights Black Spruce,™ Peppermint, Lemon, or Orange
- Starter kit essential oils: 10 drops each Peppermint, Lavender, Frankincense, and Lemon

DIY Directions: Combine essential oils into dropper bottle and swirl around to blend. Top off with Jamaican Black Castor oil and swirl to blend. This is for a single use.

Directions for Use: In a small bowl filled with hot water, place dropper bottle with top tightly in place into bowl. Let warm up for 2 minutes. Wet hair with hot water and apply warm serum all over your scalp. Use any left over to pull through the ends of hair. Tie up in a bun if you have long hair. Place shower cap over entire head and let set for 10-30 minutes. Wash thoroughly with sulfate-free shampoo.

Party Type:
Make & Take 102

SCALP SPRAY (FLAKE SUPPORT)

Ingredients:
- 4 ounce Glass Spray Bottle
- 3 ounces Distilled Water
- 10 drops each Peppermint, Lavender, Tea Tree, and Rosemary
- Starter kit essential oils: 10 drops each Peppermint, Lavender, and Frankincense

DIY Directions: Combine all essential oils into spray bottle and swirl to blend. Add distilled water and shake to mix.

Directions for Use: Spray directly onto scalp twice per day.

Party Type: Make & Take 102

ESSENTIAL OIL MAKE & TAKES by Jen O'Sullivan

SUNSCREEN (SPF 35)

Ingredients:
- 4 ounce Glass Jar
- 2 tablespoons Cocoa Butter
- 1 tablespoon Beeswax (Vegan Alternative: Candelilla Wax)
- ½ tablespoon Carrot Seed oil *(Note: Carrot Seed oil is not the same as Carrot Essential oil - There is no SPF in any essential oil.)*
- ½ tablespoon Red Raspberry Seed oil
- 1 tablespoon Zinc Oxide powder (Non Nano)
- 10 drops each Lavender and Frankincense

DIY Directions: In a double boiler, melt Cocoa Butter until melted. Turn off burner and add Carrot Seed and Red Raspberry Seed oils and blend well. Add essential oils and stir well. Slowly stir in Zinc Oxide powder while covering mouth and nose with a mask. Add a small amount at a time until it is fully blended into lotion. Use an electric mixer for several minutes to evenly distribute ingredients. Pour lotion into jar and seal tightly to let cool.

> *Note: Zinc Oxide powder is very fine. Wear gloves and mask and do not allow any to get into your lungs. Do not have small children in the room when working with Zinc Oxide. While Zinc Oxide is a natural ingredient and is non-toxic, it should not be inhaled.*

Directions for Use: Apply to exposed skin while in the sun. This sunscreen is water-resistant but not waterproof. Reapply after swimming or every 30 minutes (depending on skin burn rate) if in the water all day. Reapply every 1-2 hours or as needed.

Party Type:
Make & Take 102

ESSENTIAL OIL MAKE & TAKES by Jen O'Sullivan

TOENAIL SUPPORT

Ingredients:
- 5ml Dropper Bottle
- Jojoba oil
- 10 drops each Lavender, Oregano, and Tea Tree
- Starter kit essential oil: 20 drops each Thieves® and Lavender

DIY Directions: Combine the essential oils in the dropper bottle and swirl to blend. Add Jojoba oil and swirl to blend.

Directions for Use: Massage onto toenails twice per day.

Party Type: Make & Take 101

TOOTH POLISH

Ingredients:
- 2 ounce Glass Jar or Tube
- 4 tablespoons Baking Soda
- 1 tablespoon Raw Coconut oil (Alternative: Grapeseed oil)
- 10 drops Thieves® and 10 drops Peppermint

DIY Directions: Blend all essential oils in small clean bottle and swirl to blend. Set aside. In small bowl, blend Coconut oil and Baking Soda until mixed well. Add more or less baking soda to desired consistency. Add essential oil blend. Scoop into mini jars.

Directions for Use: Apply a pea-size amount to toothbrush. Gently brush upper teeth in a downward pulling motion from the top of your gums to the bottom of your teeth, and for your lower teeth going upward from the base of your gums up through the tips of your teeth. Brush your tongue, then spit out excess. You may rinse or leave small leftovers in mouth.

Party Type: Make & Take 101

ESSENTIAL OIL MAKE & TAKES *by Jen O'Sullivan*

UNDERARM SUPPORT

Ingredients:
- 3 tablespoons Baking Soda
- 3 tablespoons Jojoba oil
- 2 tablespoons Shea Butter (Alternative: Cocoa Butter)
- 1 tablespoon Cornstarch (Alternative: Arrowroot)
- 1 tablespoon Beeswax (Vegan Alternative: Candelilla Wax)
- 1 tablespoon Sweet Almond oil (Alternative: Grapeseed or Rosehip Seed oil)
- 20 drops Purification® and 10 drops each Lavender and Cypress essential oils
- Starter kit essential oils: 10 drops Lavender

DIY Directions: Combine Shea Butter, Beeswax, and Coconut oil in a double boiler until melted. Turn off burner. Combine Baking Soda and Cornstarch then add to mix and stir well. Add Sweet Almond oil and essential oils and blend well. Pour into containers. Let cool fully.

Directions for Use: Rub onto armpits.
> *Note: If you have never used natural deodorant, you should expect a transition period. To help support additional detox odor, use one drop of Purification® neat on armpits before you rub on Underarm Support. Detox can last 2-6 weeks.*

Party Type: Make & Take 102

UNDERARM SUPPORT (EASY)

Ingredients:
- 5ml Rollerball
- Jojoba
- 20 drops Purification® essential oil

DIY Directions: Add essential oil to rollerball and top off with Grapeseed oil.

Directions for Use: Roll onto armpits.

Party Type: Make & Take 101

ESSENTIAL OIL MAKE & TAKES by Jen O'Sullivan

WHIPPED BODY BUTTER

Ingredients:
- 2 ounce Glass Jar
- ½ cup Shea Butter
- ½ cup Raw Coconut oil (Alternative: Jojoba oil)
- ½ cup Sweet Almond oil (Alternative: Grapeseed oil)
- 1 teaspoon Vitamin E oil
- 15 drops of your favorite essential oil, such as Lavender, Peppermint, or Stress Away™

DIY Directions: Melt Shea Butter in a double boiler. Add Coconut and Sweet Almond oil and melt together, stirring constantly. Remove from heat and cool in the refrigerator for an hour to slightly set without getting hard. Remove from refrigerator, and using a hand mixer, blend well until you obtain a whipped consistency. Add essential oils to final whipping stage. Scoop into glass jar.

Directions for Use: Apply as needed.

Party Type: Make & Take 102

ESSENTIAL OIL MAKE & TAKES by Jen O'Sullivan

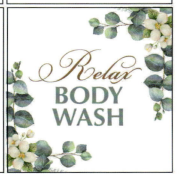

ESSENTIAL OIL MAKE & TAKES *by Jen O'Sullivan*

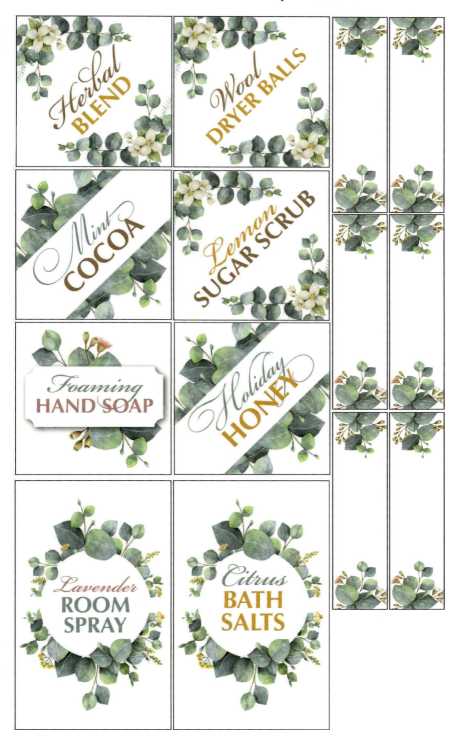

ESSENTIAL OIL MAKE & TAKES *by Jen O'Sullivan*

HOLIDAY PARTY

The holidays are a perfect time to host a holiday party. The idea is to help your friends see how easy it is to create items using their starter kit. The following 10 recipes are designed to create 10 items each using the starter kit with over half the oils left over. It is easy to create 100 gifts for all your friends using only the starter kit. Each item is designed to be under $2.50 each including the oils. You can use these as gifts for all your neighbors, teachers, and acquaintances, or join up with a few team members to each create 2-3 of them and sell them at your holiday party. Create each item using the sticker labels provided at the URL below or create color copies of the labels on the following pages.
Printable Labels: www.31oils.com/100gifts

Once made, sell each item for $5 each and include a printable recipe card so they know how you made it. That way, they can make it for themselves in the future! The follow pages contain the 100 Gift Guide or go to www.31oils. com/100gifts for linkable supplies. There are more than 10 items so you can choose which ones are right for you!

ESSENTIAL OIL MAKE & TAKES *by Jen O'Sullivan*

100 GIFTS USING THE STARTER KIT
Go to: www.31oils.com/100gifts

BREATHE ROLLERS
(Makes 10 rollers)

Ingredients:
- 5 drops each Raven™
- 10 ct. – 5ml rollers https://amzn.to/2DihVNL
- V-6™ or Dr. Adorable FCO https://amzn.to/2PE3zOg

DIY Directions: Fill bottle with carrier oil. Add essential oils. Apply roller top and screw cap. Swirl to blend well.

CANDY CANE HAND LOTION / HAND WASH
(Makes 10 sets)

Ingredients:
- 2 drops each Peppermint and Lemon
- 20 ct. – 2 ounce plastic containers https://amzn.to/2RQ0Crp
- Alaffia Lotion Unscented https://amzn.to/2PDIljz
- Alaffia Body Wash Unscented https://amzn.to/2SPVrZZ

DIY Directions: Fill container half way with base (lotion or soap). Add essential oils. Fill remainder to 2/3 full with base. Shake vigorously. Fill to top with base and shake again.

CITRUS BATH SALTS
(Makes 10)

Ingredients:
- 3-5 drops each Citrus Fresh™
- 10 ct. – 8 ounce plastic containers https://amzn.to/2T9mlvl
- Salt: online fine grain epsom salt (Saltworks) https://amzn.to/2RGx1AL
- Baking Soda (optional) https://amzn.to/2Qm2sQo

DIY Directions:
Fill bottle half way with salt, drip 3-4 drops of Citrus Fresh™ onto the salt in the middle. Fill the rest with salt. If you want to add baking soda, premix 1-2 tablespoon along with 7 ounces of salt, then add the essential oils as described above.

~ 49 ~

ESSENTIAL OIL MAKE & TAKES *by Jen O'Sullivan*

EYE SERUM
(Makes 10 serums)

Ingredients:
- 2 drops each Lavender and Frankincense
- 10 ct. – 5ml amber glass dropper bottles https://amzn.to/2TaZ2Sw
- Grapeseed oil (Dr. Adorable) https://amzn.to/2ySE8Pw
- Jamaican Black Castor oil (Cocojojo) https://amzn.to/2F4usqH

DIY Directions: Add essential oils to 5ml bottle and swirl to blend well. Fill to 1/3 full with Grapeseed oil and top of remaining 2/3 with Jamaican Black Castor oil. Swirl to blend well.

FOAMING HAND SOAP
(Makes 10 sprays)

Ingredients:
- 2 ounce Foaming Dispenser https://tinyurl.com/y6u9x992
- 6 ounces Distilled Water
- 2 tablespoons Liquid Castile Soap https://tinyurl.com/yckazl4c
- ¼ tablespoon Grapeseed oil https://amzn.to/2ySE8Pw
- 2 drops Thieves® or Lavender essential oil

DIY Directions: Combine all ingredients into dispenser making sure to leave extra room for the pump.

FOCUS ROLLER
(Makes 10 rollers)

Ingredients:
- 5 drops each PanAway®
- 10 ct. – 5ml rollers https://amzn.to/2DihVNL
- V-6™ or Dr. Adorable FCO https://amzn.to/2PE3zOg

DIY Directions: Fill bottle with carrier oil. Add essential oils. Apply roller top and screw cap. Swirl to blend well.

FRESH TOILET SPRAY
(Makes 10 sprays)

Ingredients:
- Thieves® Cleaner Packet
- 10 ct. – 2 ounce plastic spray bottles https://amzn.to/2K2xHxn

DIY Directions: Add 1/10 of the Thieves® sample packet to spray bottle. Top off with tap water. Swirl to blend well.

ESSENTIAL OIL MAKE & TAKES by Jen O'Sullivan

HERBAL BLEND
(Makes 10 jars)

Ingredients:
- 3 drops each Thieves® Vitality™
- 10 ct. – 4 ounce jars https://amzn.to/2qMhvYm
- Dandy Blend https://amzn.to/2AOxyuN

DIY Directions: Add 2 ounces of Dandy Blend to jar. Add 3 drops essential oil to the center of the mix. Top off with remaining 2 ounces of Dandy Blend.

HOLIDAY HONEY
(Makes 10 jars)

Ingredients:
- 2-3 drops each Thieves® Vitality™
- 10 ct. – 4 ounce honey jars https://amzn.to/2qMhvYm
- Organic Honey

DIY Directions: Fill container half way with honey. Add essential oils. Fill remainder with honey. Stir well with a toothpick.

LAVENDER ROOM SPRAY
(Makes 10 sprays)

Ingredients:
- 4 ounce Glass Spray Bottle
- 4 ounces Distilled Water
- 3 drops Lavender essential oil

DIY Directions: Fill bottle with distilled water, then add essential oils and shake to blend.

ESSENTIAL OIL MAKE & TAKES *by Jen O'Sullivan*

LEMON SUGAR SCRUB
(Makes 10 jars)

Ingredients:
- 10 ct. – 4 ounce jars https://amzn.to/2qMhvYm
- ¼ cup Brown Sugar
- ¼ cup Raw Cane Sugar
- 2 tablespoons Grapeseed oil https://amzn.to/2ySE8Pw
- 2 tablespoons Organic Honey (optional)
- Melted Raw Coconut Oil to desired consistency
- 10-15 drops Lemon

DIY Directions: Combine all ingredients in a bowl and blend to a wet sand consistency. It should not be crumbly, but more soupy in texture. Scoop into jar and place lid on tightly. Do not fill to the top or the oils will seep out.

MINT COCOA
(Makes 10 jars)

Ingredients:
- 3 drops each Peppermint Vitality™
- 10 ct. – 4 ounce jars https://amzn.to/2qMhvYm
- Equal Exchange Hot Cocoa Mix – Organic https://amzn.to/2JEJou8

DIY Directions: Add 2 ounces of Hot Cocoa Mix to jar. Add 3 drops essential oil to the center of the mix. Top off with remaining 2 ounces of Hot Cocoa Mix.

ESSENTIAL OIL MAKE & TAKES *by Jen O'Sullivan*

RELAX BODY LOTION / BODY WASH SET
(Makes 10 sets)

Ingredients:
- 2-3 drops each Stress Away™
- 20 ct. -2 ounce plastic containers https://amzn.to/2RQ0Crp
- Alaffia Lotion Unscented https://amzn.to/2PDIljz
- Alaffia Body Wash Unscented https://amzn.to/2SPVrZZ

DIY Directions: Fill container half way with base (lotion or soap). Add essential oils. Fill remainder to 2/3 full with base. Shake vigorously. Fill to top with base and shake again.

ROLLERS
(Makes as many rollers as you like)

Ingredients:
- 5 drops each essential oil of choice
    Examples:
        Happy Tummy: DiGize™
        Party On: PanAway®
        Happy Days: Citrus Fresh™ or Lemon
        Holiday Perfume: Thieves®
        Brainiac: 3 drops Valor® and 2 drops Frankincense
        Calm Down: 3 drops Peace & Calming and 2 drops Lavender
- 10 ct. – 5ml rollers https://amzn.to/2DihVNL
- V-6™ or Dr. Adorable FCO https://amzn.to/2PE3zOg

DIY Directions: Fill bottle with carrier oil. Add essential oils. Apply roller top and screw cap. Swirl to blend well.

WOOL DRYER BALLS SET
(Makes 10 sets)

Ingredients:
- 20 ct. Dryer Balls https://amzn.to/2RPz0m4
- 10 ct. Lavender sachet samples
- Cute gift bags or sacks

DIY Directions: Place two dryer balls along with one Lavender sachet into a bag and tie with a ribbon.

ESSENTIAL OIL MAKE & TAKES *by Jen O'Sullivan*

FINAL THOUGHTS

It can be very empowering to make your own products and be 100 percent confident of your ingredients. It's even better that your products have ingredients that you can actually read and pronounce. (Jojoba oil is pronounced *Hohoba*, in case you wondered.) I am a busy mom who really just wants to hang out with my family. I limit any and all extra busy work in my life as much as possible. So when it comes to making my own products, I want them to be quick and easy.

This book contains my quick, easy, and sometimes dirty recipes ('cuz let's be real, I am a mess in the kitchen) that are so much healthier for me and my family—plus, most are pennies on the dollar from what I would have spent at the store. Okay, so the *Whipped Body Butter* takes a little more time and energy, so, for that reason, it is only in my house about once a year. You know, the time of year I start to feel like "Suzy Homemaker" and I get the gumption to go on a hunt for my hand mixer. I'm usually hoping to find BOTH beaters, but I've been known to make use of just one in a pinch.

The reality is we are all busy, but our health should not take a back seat. I always say, "When mom is down, we all are down." Somehow my house just seems to completely disintegrate when I am not well. These chemical-free products will help eliminate the majority of the endocrine disruptors in your life. Did you catch that!? Endocrine disruptors! They are all around you, even *right now* as you read this.

What are endocrine disruptors? First let's understand what your endocrine system is. Your endocrine system is the engine for your entire hormonal system. Your hormones are like your soil. If a plant's soil is depleted and bad, the whole plant looks terrible and produces nothing. So if your endocrine system is being disrupted, YOU will look terrible and YOU will produce nothing. Yikes!

Now, moving on to those sneaky little disruptors. I said they are all around you, and I am not joking. Not even a little bit. The ink on this very page you are reading is a synthetic and could cause a disruption to your endocrine system if you are around publishing ink enough. (Rest assured, as a reader of books you are fine, but if you worked in a print house, you could experience some hormone issues long term.) Here are just a few to demonstrate the insidiousness of these disruptors.

KNOWN ENDOCRINE DISRUPTORS

Household cleaners, pharmaceuticals, phytoestrogens found in soy, bovine protein, household dust (huge), plastic storage containers... plus, there are many hidden endocrine disruptors found in just about everything from kids' toys to nail polish, antiperspirants, shampoos

~ 54 ~

ESSENTIAL OIL MAKE & TAKES *by Jen O'Sullivan*

and conditioners with parabens and sulfates, body wash, toothpaste, lotions, sunscreens, shaving gel, cosmetics, plastic bottles that contain BPA, Teflon® pans and baking molds, tampons, laundry detergent, dryer sheets, fabric softeners, dishwasher detergent, mattresses, memory foam, fire retardants, air fresheners, synthetic fragrances, vinyl shower curtains, electric blankets, anti-bacterial hand soap containing triclosan, insect repellent, phthalates found in so many things it is scary: fragrances, shampoo, air fresheners, new car smell, steering wheel, vinyl flooring—the list goes on and on! You can see a full list of chemicals to avoid at www.ewg.org or the EWG app.

What's a girl to do? Go back through this book and earmark every single page with the recipes you need to make! They are really not that hard, and you can start replacing all of your chemically yuckiness one product at a time. Consider this: if you simply tackled one recipe per week, you could replace over 50 items in your house in a year! They each only take around 10 minutes or less to make, so time is not an excuse. You can slowly build up your supply base by purchasing ingredients here and there and then use them throughout the year, so money is also not an excuse (except for the *Sunscreen*, that is a bit pricey but WAY worth the chemical crap storm you are avoiding from store-bought brands). Remember, these products will actually SAVE you money. Here are some comparisons of my own savings.

Dove® Deodorant	$4.39	vs. $1.50
Tom's® Toothpaste	$3.99	vs. $2.80
Neutrogena® Toner	$7.49	vs. $2.40
Neutrogena® Makeup Remover	$6.49	vs. $2.60
Neutrogena® Moisturizer	$9.99	vs. $5.80
Neutrogena® Eye Cream	$17.99	vs. $6.50
Paul Mitchell® Smoothing	$20.99	vs. $8.90
Windex®	$3.14	vs. $2.10
Febreze® Air Effects	$5.09	vs. $1.70
Beard Guyz™ Beard Balm	$14.99	vs. $6.40
Bourdeaux's® Paste	$7.99	vs. $2.50
	$102.54	**$43.20**

THAT'S A SAVINGS OF $59.34! Yes please!

I hope you are empowered and energized to clean up your home and lifestyle! Reach out to the person who gave you this book and make things together! Get a group of ladies to go in together to split the costs on bulk items to make it even more inexpensive and fun. Enjoy this journey, and I wish you all the success for a more happy and healthful life!

ESSENTIAL OIL MAKE & TAKES *by Jen O'Sullivan*

INGREDIENT LIST

- ☐ Almonds, ground
- ☐ Aloe Vera Gel
- ☐ Aloe Vera Juice
- ☐ Apple Cider Vinegar
- ☐ Arrowroot
- ☐ Avocado
- ☐ Azuki Beans
- ☐ Baking Soda (Not Baking Powder)
- ☐ Beeswax Pellets
- ☐ Beeswax Sheets
- ☐ Brown Sugar
- ☐ Calcium Carbonate Powder
- ☐ Candelilla Wax
- ☐ Cane Sugar
- ☐ Carrot Seed Oil (Organic)
- ☐ Castile Soap – Dr. Bronner's
- ☐ Castile Soap – Natural Way Organics
- ☐ Citric Acid
- ☐ Copaiba Vanilla Conditioner
- ☐ Cocoa Butter
- ☐ Cocoa Powder (Unsweetened)
- ☐ Coconut Oil (Organic, raw)
- ☐ Cornstarch
- ☐ Distilled Water
- ☐ Egg White
- ☐ Essential Oils
- ☐ Everclear® Grain Alcohol
- ☐ Food Coloring

- ☐ Grapeseed Oil (Organic)
- ☐ Honey (Organic)
- ☐ Jamaican Black Castor Oil
- ☐ Jojoba Oil (Organic)
- ☐ Lavender Buds (Organic)
- ☐ Mango Butter
- ☐ Massage Oils
- ☐ Molasses
- ☐ Oats, Gluten Free (Quick Oats)
- ☐ Pumpkin Seed Oil (Organic)
- ☐ Sweet Almond Oil (Organic)
- ☐ Red Raspberry Oil (Organic)
- ☐ Rosehip Seed Oil (Organic)
- ☐ Rubbing Alcohol
- ☐ Salt – Dead Sea
- ☐ Salt – Epsom
- ☐ Salt – Pink Himalayan
- ☐ Saponified Coconut Oil Liquid Soap
- ☐ Shea Butter
- ☐ Sugar – Brown
- ☐ Sugar – Cane, Raw
- ☐ Sugar - White
- ☐ Vegetable Glycerin
- ☐ Vitamin E Oil
- ☐ White Vinegar
- ☐ Witch Hazel
- ☐ Zinc Oxide Powder

ESSENTIAL OIL MAKE & TAKES *by Jen O'Sullivan*

RESOURCES

Brands:
- Cocojojo
- Dr. Adorable
- Dr. Bronner's
- Liquid Gold
- Mary Tyler Naturals
- Natural Way Organics

Retailers:
- Amazon
- eBay
- Life Science Publishing
- My Oily Habit
- Trader Joe's
- Many others!

EQUIPMENT LIST

- Coffee Grinder
- Electric Mixer
- Funnel
- Measuring Cups
- Measuring Spoons
- Mixing Bowl
- Molds
- Pipettes
- Pyrex Bowls
- Ramekin, Small
- Stainless Steel Pot
- Large Lid

SUPPLY LIST
Obtain glass when available.

- Atomizer, Fragrance
- Candle Wick
- Containers, Small
- Cotton Rounds
- Dropper Bottles
- Fabric Glue
- Foaming Soap Dispenser
- Jars, Glass
- Pump Bottle
- Quilting Squares
- Rollerballs
- Spice Shaker
- Spray Bottle, Glass
- Tubes, Lip Balm size
- Tubes, Deodorant size
- Water Jug, Glass

ESSENTIAL OIL MAKE & TAKES *by Jen O'Sullivan*

HOW TO HOST A MAKE & TAKE PARTY

If you are an essential oil distributor, hosting a Make & Take essential oil party can be exciting and fun, yet completely overwhelming and very hard on your pocketbook. It is easy to go crazy making what we think will "wow" our guests by Martha-ing the party to death! You know the drill: You clean the house top to bottom. You create the most delicious oil-infused food, goodies, and treats, as well as have lavender spa lemonade that is to die for!

Forget about dull make and take items! You go all out by coming up with six amazing DIY Make & Take stations all throughout your kitchen, dining room, and living room. You even have a great decorating station, complete with the cutest DIY labels, pens, and washi tape. The guests arrive and proceed to have the most fun at an in-home party that they can remember.

It is a hit! You all socialize and laugh hysterically, make great oily projects, decorate them all to perfection, and everyone leaves with amazing products to try… and NO ONE buys any oils!

The sad reality is that this happens more often than not. Make & Takes, while very fun, are not IPAs (Income Producing Activities). There are two types of people who come to a Make & Take: current customers and potential customers. You will want to strategically invite your guests so you know which type of Make & Take party to throw.

For ease of describing the parties, the Make & Take parties for newbies who are not yet customers will be referred to as "Make & Take 101." For current customers, these parties will be referred to as "Make & Take 102." The concept is to create a fun party for new people as an Basics of Oils event combined with an easy introduction Make & Take that only uses oils in the in the starter oils kit.

~ 58 ~

ESSENTIAL OIL MAKE & TAKES *by Jen O'Sullivan*

Your goal is to make it super simple and easy. Do not overdo it. Resist the urge! For your current customers, you would also make it simple, but create a customer appreciation class where you teach a more advanced projects and you introduce oils outside the starter kit.

This book contains some of the most loved Make & Take projects and will help you determine which type of party they are best suited for. You will also notice the projects are made with oils from the starter kit, or there will be a line item that suggests which starter kit oils to use as alternatives.

All item sizes are based on personal use. It is suggested you use the smallest size available. For instance, instead of using a 15ml dropper bottle, cut the recipe in thirds and use a 5ml, or even smaller by using a 2ml. Make sure the cost for all items totals less than $3 each with all supplies included.

For the Make & Take 102, your customers would bring their own oils and you would introduce new oils for them to smell (but not use). Teach them how to add the new oils to their monthly order after class.

If you would rather allow them to use your oils, it is very important that you make smaller sample-size batches and charge accordingly. Making full-size eye serums for everyone will get very expensive, and the goal is to have them purchase their own oils to make the project again after class.

Enjoy making all the fun items in this book! Check out the full party script for you to use on the next page! Have fun!

~ 59 ~

ESSENTIAL OIL MAKE & TAKES *by Jen O'Sullivan*

MAKE & TAKE PARTY SCRIPT

The following are instructions on how to host a successful Make & Take class. You can find more details and information on hosting a class or party in the book "Essentially Driven."

• Invite 4 times as many people as you would like to attend.

• Personally invite each person 1-2 weeks before the event. Do not send out a group email or e-vite. A personal phone call, text message, or email is good depending on the person.

> Sample invite: *Hi Amy! Several of us ladies are getting together at my place next week on (date and time) to make candles and to chat about essential oils. Can you join us? I love candles but hate the ones from the store because they give me such a headache. We are going to make toxic free candles that are super easy. Let me know if you can make it so I can order the right amount of supplies!*

• If the person says they can come, leave out some information so you can have multiple connection points as reminders.
Example connection points:

> *1.* Four days before, ask if they have any friends they would like to bring so you can have enough supplies for the group project.
> *2.* Two days before, give them your address.
> *3.* One day before, share that you are very excited about the party and ask them if they are able to come a little early to help you set up. Purposefully leave items unfinished such as sprucing up the bathroom, setting up the diffuser, or helping put out some snacks. Every guest should be tasked with something to help you in the set up of your party. This ensures they show up, and are on time.
> *4.* Day of, let them know something pertinent to the area such as where to park or how to access your gate or front door.

1. Get the party started with a DIY Make & Take project. This will allow guests who arrive late to not miss the important class part. Use one of the Oil 101 projects in this book.

2. After the project is complete, either continue in the room you are in, or gather your guests to the main presentation room, such as your living room if you were working in your kitchen. Welcome your guests again and share a little about you and why you got into oils. Tell a short 3-5 minute testimonial about how oils have changed your life and tie it into the Make & Take item you just made.

3. Briefly introduce the kit. Share the price: both retail and wholesale.
4. Go over the basics of essential oils in under 60 seconds.

ESSENTIAL OIL MAKE & TAKES *by Jen O'Sullivan*

Basics of Oils Sample: Essential oils are the life-force of plants. They help the plant to regulate itself and add health and overall wellness. These oils can work in much the same way for us. There are three ways to use essential oils: aromatic, topical, and internal. It takes 20 minutes for essential oils to reach every cell in your body from the time you apply them. There are around 40 trillion cells in our bodies, and one drop of essential oil contains over 40 million trillion molecules! This means every single cell in our body, in 20 minutes, is covered by one million essential oil molecules.

5. Go over each oil in the starter kit and pass the oil around as you discuss it so they can smell it. This is the best time to tell your stories.

6. Share why the brand is different from all other brands. Cover the guarantee and testing processes (the brand comparison chart from 31oils.com is excellent for this!) Do a smell test using three oils (optional). Use Peppermint and two other companies, such as a major competitor and one that you can buy in a grocery store. All of them should be covered up so you do not disclose who the other brands are. This becomes a wonderful opportunity to share the difference between how oils are processed and why the smell can help you know the difference. Share the "Quality Chart" found in "Essentially Driven" and "Live Well" books.

7. Go over what else comes in the starter kit.

8. Ask happily and in a heartfelt way if anyone would like to buy a starter kit, host a party, or join your team! Share briefly what the business has done for you and how you would love to help them host their first party. Then tell them, "First things first, I want you to fall head over heels in love with your oils, so let's order your kit!" Ask for the sale. Don't just wrap it up and say goodnight. Don't peter out with a Q&A session. Get oils into their home!

9. End on time and don't forget to laugh and have fun. Do not do anything over-produced at parties. Simple, pretty, and fun is best! Don't go crazy stressing yourself out about it. Think of it like a fun friends' night out. The more over the top you make your parties and classes, the harder it will be for others to envision themselves doing it. You want people to say, "Wow, I could totally do this!"

10. For those who did not buy a kit, find out why and then follow up. Be friendly and continue to share your love and passion for the oils and why you know they will love them too!

11. Do it again and again and again! Practice makes perfect, and while classes do not need to be perfect, your nerves will be more settled the more you teach.

ESSENTIAL OIL MAKE & TAKES by Jen O'Sullivan

ADDITIONAL EDUCATION

BOOKS BY JEN available at 31oils.com and Amazon

- "The Supplements Desk Reference"
- "Wellness" (the Essential Oil book)
- "Purpose" (the Thieves® book)
- "Abundance" (the NingXia Red® book)
- "The Essential oil Truth: The Facts Without The Hype"
- "French Aromatherapy: Essential oil Recipes & Usage Guide"
- "VITALITY: The Young Living® Lifestyle"
- "The RECIPE Book with Jen O'Sullivan"
- "Essentially Driven"
- "Live Well"

ONLINE EDUCATION

- Intro to Oils: www.vitalityedu.com/oils
- 12 Day eCourse: www.vitalityedu.com/subscribe
- Wellness course: www.vitalityedu.com/wellness
- VLC Certification: www.vitalityedu.com/vlc
- Facebook: www.facebook.com/jenosullivanauthor
- Facebook: www.facebook.com/groups/thehumanbody
- Archive: www.vitalityedu.com/thehumanbody
- YouTube: www.youtube.com/c/jenstips
- Instagram: @jenauthor

EDUCATIONAL TOOLS

Books and Brochures: www.31oils.com

Mobile App:

- The EO Bar

ESSENTIAL OIL MAKE & TAKES *by Jen O'Sullivan*

AUTHOR BIOGRAPHY

Jen O'Sullivan believes that getting to the root of the problem is vital to full health and restoration and utilizes a whole-body system approach of care with her students and customers. She has been an essential oil user since 2007, and absolutely adores helping people on their path to wellness. She is known for her up-front and to-the-point education style. Jen has studied health and nutrition since 2007 and has the ability to take complicated information and share it in a way that makes it easy to understand. Jen is certified in French Medicinal Aromatherapy through the School for Aromatic Studies and has been a professional educator since 1999, at both the collegiate and high school levels. She is lovingly known as "The oil lady to the oil ladies" and is the author of eight Amazon best-sellers. She has developed one of the largest and most comprehensive essential oil education and recipe usage apps on the market today called "The EO Bar". Her online education group of over a quarter of a million oil enthusiasts called "The Human Body and Essential oils" (www.Facebook.com/groups/TheHumanBody) is her main group where she teaches proper usage and safety with essential oils. She also has a full on-line educational school called Vitality EDU (www.VitalityEDU.com) where she offers certification courses as well as free and tuition based education. Jen lives in Southern California with her husband and high school sweetheart Tim and their son Jacob, and fur-baby, Dash the min pin.

You can hear Jen's story at www.VitalityEDU.com/jen

Be blessed!

ESSENTIAL OIL MAKE & TAKES *by Jen O'Sullivan*

PERSONAL RECIPES